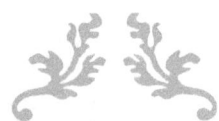

# PIRACETAM

*50 THINGS YOU NEED TO KNOW ABOUT BRAIN BOOSTING NOOTROPICS*

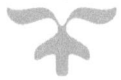

LEROY JENKINS

# Table of Contents

INTRODUCTION...................................................................................................2

**Chapter 1** ........................................................................................................6

   History Of Piracetam........................................................................................6

**Chapter 2** ........................................................................................................7

   Uses Of Piracetam...........................................................................................7

**Chapter 3** ........................................................................................................9

   Benefits Of Piracetam .....................................................................................9

**Chapter 4** ......................................................................................................12

   Methods To Use.............................................................................................12

**Chapter 5** ......................................................................................................14

   Toxicity, Side Effects, Availability, Better Alternative To Piracetam .....................14

**Chapter 6** ......................................................................................................18

   50 Things You Need To Know About Brain Boosting Nootropics............................18

**Chapter 7** ......................................................................................................44

   What Are Nootropics? ....................................................................................44

**Conclusion** ....................................................................................................52

# INTRODUCTION

Nootropics, or smart drugs, are natural or synthetic substances intended to improve your mental performance.

Piracetam is considered the first nootropic drug of its kind. It can be purchased online or in health food stores and comes in both capsule and powder form. It's a popular synthetic derivative of the neurotransmitter gamma-Aminobutyric acid (GABA), a chemical messenger that helps slow down activity in your nervous system.

Piracetam has been around since the 1960s and is regarded as a pioneer "smart drug." It enjoys a popular, international following, its record as a treatment for cognitive disorders is impressive, and scientific exams haven't flagged any dangerous side effects. But is Piracetam truly the intelligence booster many of us eagerly want?

Despite decades of global drug research, the field of cognitive enhancement remains unknown amongst the general public and conspicuously absent in consideration of public health policy. Mention the word 'nootropic' to the average person on the street in the developed world, and the likely response is a blank look with perhaps a query about tropical fruit. Comparatively small numbers of people are aware of nootropic substances or their growing usage.

The mildest member of the 'Racetam' family, Piracetam is often billed as a 'beginners drug' for nootropics due to its safety. This explains its prevalence amongst college students seeking an extra boost for exams, as well as experimenters looking for an easy opening into this expanding market.

As a detoxifying agent, Piracetam is used to treat the damaging effects of alcoholism by enhancing oxygen utilization in the brain, which rapidly degenerates during alcohol consumption. It also impedes the destruction of neurons in the hippocampus during the period immediately following alcohol withdrawal. Piracetam also counteracts the cumulative effects of other toxic substances by preventing the hypoxia that occurs as a result of tobacco smoke and reversing the short term memory loss associated with marijuana usage.

Evidence exists for its use as a metabolism booster. Its hypoxia-preventing ◻ualities can improve athletic performance at high-altitudes and substantially reduce fatigue, and prolong the lives of rats and mice suffering from severe hypoxia.

Piracetam also protects the cardiovascular system by improving blood circulation to the brain, and may thereby alleviate cerebral insufficiency. It is believed to counteract the effects of Atherosclerosis and Raynaud's disease, again by preventing hypoxia. Due to its enhancement of oxygen functioning in the brain, Piracetam can improve the after-care for strokes, and serve as a long-term treatment for clotting, coagulation, and vasospastic disorders such as Deep-Vein Thrombosis.

Perhaps more importantly, it offers a host of positive effects for the nervous system. It's been effective in treating cognitive disorders of cerebrovascular and traumatic origins, although it's superior at lowering depression and anxiety than it is at improving memory. Clinical studies have demonstrated Piracetam's benefits in treating neuro-diseases such as Alzheimer's and Dementia by improving alertness and memory function while reducing confusion and alleviating paranoia.

This nootropic has even been used to improve the hearing of persons who have sudden deafness and hearing loss, alleviate the learning disorders associated with attention deficit disorder, and to mitigate the effects of some sleep disorders. There are suggestions that for some autistic conditions the drug has been used to great effect in improving motor development, mental development, speech, emotional development, academic achievement and EEG, particularly in Down's syndrome patients. It may also improve most aspects of mental function, including speed and accuracy of reading, short-term memory and verbal memory, in Dyslexia patients and Epileptics.

All of this attests to Piracetam's reliability as a drug of obvious medical worth. But what effects, if any, does it have upon comparatively healthy minds?

In elderly test groups, it has produced □uite dramatic results. A study of elderly drivers found that after ingesting Piracetam for 6 weeks, the drivers demonstrated significantly better performance than the placebo group, in overall reaction capacity, perception and orientation. Of particular interest is the finding that the test-subjects who had scored less than 80% in the pre-test improved without exception in the retest after treatment with Piracetam.

Studies like this are supported by animal trials which show that the treatment of mice is associated with improved mitochondrial function in dissociated brain cells, with significant benefit mainly seen in aged animals.

It seems reasonable to assume cogent positives for adults at large, who use Piracetam as a supplement. On the neuronal level, Piracetam modulates neurotransmission in a range of transmitter systems (including cholinergic and glutamatergic), has neuroprotective and anticonvulsant properties and improves neuroplasticity. Studies suggest that it improves attention span in normal, healthy humans, and enhances creativity by increasing communication between the two hemispheres of the brain.

There's also the possibility that healthy adults using Piracetam can increase certain aspects of their intelligence, such as memory. This is achieved by increasing the synthesis of proteins responsible for the formation of new memories, enhancing learning abilities by influencing the cerebral cortex, protecting against memory loss from physical injury and chemical poisoning, rejuvenating aged and damaged neurons, and elevating spatial awareness.

# Chapter 1

## History Of Piracetam

Piracetam is a nootropic drug in the racetams group, with chemical name 2-oxo-1-pyrrolidine acetamide. It shares the same 2-oxo-pyrrolidone base structure with pyroglutamic acid and is a cyclic derivative of the neurotransmitter γ-aminobutyric acid (GABA). However, its mechanism of action differs from that of endogenous GABA. Piracetam has neuroprotective and anticonvulsant properties and is reported to improve neural plasticity. Its efficacy is documented in cognitive disorders and dementia, vertigo, cortical myoclonus, dyslexia, and sickle cell anemia, although the clinical application in these conditions is not yet established. Piracetam has effects on the vascular system by reducing erythrocyte adhesion to vascular endothelium, hinder vasospasm and facilitate microcirculation.

Originally marketed by UCB Pharma in 1971, Piracetam was the first nootropic drug to modulate cognitive function without causing sedation or stimulation. It is not approved for any medical or dietary use by the FDA. In the U.K., Piracetam is prescribed mainly for myoclonus but is used off-label for other conditions such as learning difficulties in children, memory loss or other cognitive defects in the elderly, and sickle-cell vaso-occlusive crises. Evidence to support its use for many conditions is unclear.

# Chapter 2

## Uses Of Piracetam

Piracetam is said to act as a nootropic, a class of drugs designed to enhance memory and boost cognitive function. In alternative medicine, it's thought that piracetam can help increase brain function by promoting communication between the left and right hemispheres of the brain.

Also, piracetam is purported to treat or **prevent the following health problems:**

- Alzheimer's disease
- Anxiety
- Central nervous system disorders (such as epilepsy)
- Deep vein thrombosis
- Depression
- Vertigo
- Stroke

Piracetam is also said to slow up the aging process and promote recovery from alcoholism.

**Therapeutic use of Piracetam**

Piracetam has been used in medicine for many years, with positive effects on various disease processes and mental disorders. It counteracts memory impairment, learning disabilities, disorders of mating and remembrance, and issues related to adapting to the new environment and social adjustment.

It is used in the treatment of cognitive disorders in dementia, pathological involuntary movements (myoclonic) of cortical origin, dizziness, dyslexia (specific learning difficulties in reading and writing, and the treatment of attention deficit hyperactivity disorder (ADHD).

In general, piracetam increases the consumption of glucose and oxygen in the brain that precedes cognitive improvement (these actions are global - they do not favor only "some" brain regions) and is more significant in people with cognitive impairment). It also has proven research into the benefits of rehabilitation after stroke - much faster restores brain function and activates larger areas of work.

# Chapter 3

## Benefits Of Piracetam

So far, scientific support for the benefits of piracetam is limited. **Here's a look at several study findings on the potential benefits:**

- **Stroke:** For a report published in the Cochrane Database of Systematic Reviews in 2012, investigators analyzed the available research on the use of piracetam among stroke patients. The study's authors note that piracetam can help protect against the formation of blood clots and shield nerve cells from injury or breakdown, which could benefit stroke patients. However, looking at data from three clinical trials (involving a total of 1,002 patients), the report's authors found no evidence that piracetam can help improve functioning or reduce mortality in people who have experienced a stroke.

- **Cognitive Impairment:** Piracetam may benefit older adults who have dementia or cognitive impairment, according to a 2002 report published in Dementia & Geriatric Cognitive Disorders. Analyzing the results of 19 previously published studies, the report's authors found that piracetam was superior to placebo in the treatment of older adults with cognitive impairment.

- **Central Nervous System Disorders:** A report published in the journal Drugs in 2010 suggests that piracetam shows promise in the treatment of central nervous system disorders. Sizing up the available research on piracetam for central nervous system disorders, the report's authors determined that piracetam may aid in the treatment of depression, anxiety, myoclonus epilepsy, and tardive dyskinesia (a type of neurological disorder).

- **Supporting Short-Term Memory And Learning Capacity:** One study found the use of piracetam over 14 days resulted in significantly better word recall and improvements in short-term working memory.

Piracetam has also been tested among children with dyslexia. While study results have been somewhat mixed and hard to replicate, certain studies have found that it led to improvements in reading rate, verbal learning and comprehension when taken daily for up to eight weeks.

- **Mood Enhancement:** When it comes to mood improvement, more research about piracetam's effects is needed. A lot of anecdotal evidence exists, stating it may help support mood stabilization and mental health, concentration, verbal intelligence, energy, motivation and more — but so far, the scientific proof has been limited. Recent research also shows it can work as an antidepressant, improve the brain's "reward properties" and reduce the negative effects of drug/alcohol withdrawal on the central nervous system.

- **Preventing Blood Clots:** Research shows that piracetam may be useful following cardiovascular trauma because it helps to stop blood clots from forming, similar to aspirin. It's also been shown to have protective effects in patients undergoing coronary artery bypass surgery. Additionally, piracetam affects blood flow by boosting circulation and helping to prevent blood vessels from constricting.

Because it can help prevent blood clots from developing, the drug is being investigated as a way to lower the risk for strokes. It has been shown in some, but not all, studies to help with stroke recovery, including language function. However, because of inconclusive research findings, it's still not recommended that patients recovering from acute ischemic stroke take piracetam routinely.

- **Protecting Against Oxidative Stress:** There's evidence that piracetam can increase membrane fluidity in the brain and reduce rigidity associated with oxidative and lipid stress. Piracetam seems to help normalize fluidity and mitochondrial function, both of which suffer when the brain is impacted by free radicals, inflammation, injury and aging. Researchers have also associated a loss of normal fluidity in the mitochondria with states of cognitive decline.

# Chapter 4

## Methods To Use

Piracetam should be used in two or three divided doses during the day.

- The standard dose of piracetam for children during ADHD treatment is between 40-100mg per kilogram body weight.
- For adults, it is recommended to take 1000-1200 mg 2-3 times a day due to the 4-8 hours half-life.
- Cognitive disorders are treated with a maximum daily dose of 2.4 g. The effects of the administration of the preparation are not apparent until after prolonged use.

Piracetam does not cause physical dependence. It can increase physical fitness and sex drive. Do not use in the evening because it can cause problems falling asleep.

### Which Supplements To Use With Piracetam

If your doctor has directed you to use this medication, your doctor or pharmacist may already be aware of any possible drug interactions and may be monitoring you for them. Do not start, stop, or change the dosage of any medicine before checking with your doctor, health care provider or pharmacist first.

Piracetam has no known severe or serious interactions with other drugs.

Moderate interactions of **piracetam include:**

- cilostazol
- clopidogrel
- dipyridamole
- eptifibatide
- prasugrel
- ticlopidine
- tirofiban

Mild interactions of **piracetam include:**

- levothyroxine
- liothyronine
- thyroid desiccated

This information does not contain all possible interactions or adverse effects. Therefore, before using this product, tell your doctor or pharmacist of all the products you use. Keep a list of all your medications with you, and share this information with your doctor and pharmacist. Check with your health care professional or doctor for additional medical advice, or if you have health ☐uestions, concerns or for more information about this medicine.

# Chapter 5

## Toxicity, Side Effects, Availability, Better Alternative To Piracetam

Piracetam does not appear to be acutely toxic at the doses used in human studies. The LD50 for oral consumption in humans has not been determined. The LD50 is 5.6 g/kg for rats and 20 g/kg for mice, indicating extremely low acute toxicity. For comparison, in rats, the LD50 of vitamin C is 12 g/kg, and the LD50 of table salt is 3 g/kg.

**Side Effects**

Common side effects of **piracetam include:**

- Diarrhea
- Weight gain
- Drowsiness
- Insomnia
- Nervousness
- Depression
- Muscle spasm
- Hyperactivity
- Rash

This document does not contain all possible side effects, and others may occur. Check with your physician for additional information about side effects.

## Availability

Piracetam is sold under a wide variety of brand names worldwide. Popular trade names for piracetam in Europe are Nootropil and Lucetam, among many others. In Argentina, it is made by GlaxoSmithKline S.A. laboratories and sold under the trade name of Noostan (800 mg or 1200 mg). In Venezuela and Ecuador, piracetam is produced by Laboratorios Farma S.A. and sold under the brand name Breinox. In Mexico, it is produced by UCB de Mexico, and sold under the brand name of Nootropil. Other names include Nootropil in the United States, Europe, Brazil, Hong Kong, India, and Mexico; Lucetam, Oikamid, Smart, Geratam, and Biotropil in Europe and Brazil; Neurobasal in Colombia; Breinox in Ecuador and Venezuela; Cerecetam in India; Stimulan in Egypt; and Nocetan in Latin America.

## Better Alternatives To Piracetam

Rather than experimenting with a drug that is still under investigation and not necessarily effective for most healthy adults, try these nootropic alternatives **to piracetam instead:**

- **Omega-3 fish oils** — Studies show omega-3s can support cognitive function by helping reduce inflammation, preserve memory and protect against depression and Alzheimer's disease. In addition to, or instead of supplementing, you can obtain omega-3s from wild-caught fish like salmon, sardines, tuna, mackerel and herring.

- **Medicinal mushrooms, such as Chaga, cordyceps and reishi** — These "functional fungi" have been shown in studies to help support cognitive function and fight cognitive impairment in older adults due to their antioxidant properties and ability to increase resilience during times of stress, including by balancing hormones like cortisol.

- **Adaptogen herbs, such as ashwagandha, astralagus and Rhodiola** — These herbs are effective at improving stress response, lowering blood corticosterone levels (a stress hormone), fighting fatigue, supporting the adrenals and creating positive alterations in the neurotransmitter system of the brain.

- **Green tea extract** — When used appropriately, green tea and other sources of natural caffeine can have mood-enhancing effects, fight inflammation and oxidative stress and increase alertness and productivity.

- **Ginseng** — Ginseng is another herb that can improve calmness, some aspects of working memory and performance and provide protection against fatigue and stress.

- **Gingko Biloba** — Gingko has been shown to have anti-inflammatory, antioxidant, platelet-forming and circulation-boosting effects.

Piracetam is a synthetic nootropic that may boost mental performance. Its positive effects on the brain seem more apparent in older adults, as well as people with mental impairment, dementia, or learning disorders, such as dyslexia.

That said, very few studies on piracetam exist, and most of the research is dated, so new research is needed before it can be recommended. Piracetam is relatively safe for most people. Still, if you're taking medication or have any medical disorders, speak to your healthcare provider before trying this drug.

# Chapter 6

## 50 Things You Need To Know About Brain Boosting Nootropics

The hottest drug right now is designed to make you smarter. Nootropics sometimes called "smart drugs," are synthetic compounds that have been credited with everything from keeping users focused on making people rich. But there are still a lot of unknowns surrounding nootropics, and much of the evidence in existence is more anecdotal than scientific.

On a basic level, nootropics modify the supply of enzymes, hormones, and neurotransmitters in the brain. But the exact definition of the drugs and their effects can be difficult to pin down since nootropic drugs and nootropic drug combinations (known as "stacks") interact in different ways with the brain and body. Some have been available for years as prescription drugs, but many can be obtained without a prescription.

Nootropics have also been the source of controversy. While there is an entire faction of users who credit nootropics for helping them lead happier, more productive lives, there is another faction that encourages extreme caution with these substances until more definitive information is known. Before you start using nootropics, **it is important to know these 50 things:**

## 1. Quality is important.

Research published in the Journal of the American Medical Association shows that in the last nine years, unapproved pharmaceutical agents were found in 776 different dietary supplements. This study emphasized the fact that □uality ingredients and manufacturing is important. Often, nootropic ingredients are purchased on the open market, and one cannot trace their source and verify the purity of the ingredients. Giving people peace of mind about □uality and purity was an important factor when Neutein was developed. This is why Neutein only contains patented all-natural plant-based ingredients where we can track the journey from seed to field to capsule. Neutein is also manufactured in an FDA inspected facility that is GMP certified.

## 2. Not all nootropics are researched in healthy people.

Brains are all different. Especially the brains of healthy individuals compared to people that may already be suffering from cognitive decline. Because there is considerable interest in improving the health of failing brains, more research goes into nootropics that might help people in those populations, which doesn't always translate into supplements working in a healthy brain. For example, a couple of studies show that when people take 400 mg of the nootropic alpha-GPC three times a day with mild to moderate Alzheimer's disease, it can slightly improve cognitive function after three months of daily use. You might hear that alpha-GPC would work for you (perhaps a younger person with no cognitive decline), but unfortunately, there is no evidence to support that, despite tons of alpha-GPC being sold to improve mental function. Before you take a nootropic, make sure science says it will work for you.

### 3. Some nootropics make you jittery or give you anxiety.

Nootropics can enhance your mental function and performance in a variety of different ways. Many nootropics, like caffeine or yohimbine, are stimulants. They can increase your heart rate and level of alertness by stimulating your nervous system. Unfortunately, this can also increase anxiety. One interesting fact about caffeine is that it not only increases your reaction time but also can decrease the accuracy of your reaction. On the other hand, research shows that Neutein increases both reaction time and accuracy of reaction time, while not being a stimulant that increases your heart rate, makes you jittery, nor increases the feeling of anxiety.

### 4. There is no one-size-fits-all nootropic.

Nootropics, as a class of supplements/drugs, covers a wide range of functions ranging from improving motivation to creativity to focus and attention. This means you aren't likely to find a nootropic that does everything. It is important to determine what benefit you would like to have and then find a product that supports it. For example, if you would like to improve your focus and attention, Neutein contains antioxidants that have been shown in three different studies to do this. But if you would like to enhance your creativity, then l-theanine is the supplement that may be able to help with that.

### 5. How much you take matters.

One of the biggest areas where people make mistakes with nootropics (or supplements in general) is with how much they take. If you have a headache and take ibuprofen, you know that you need to take a certain amount for it to be effective. The same is true for nootropics. Just because you are taking a supplement that contains ashwagandha (a herb purported to help with stress management) that doesn't mean you are going to reap the benefits. Research shows that you need 200 mg, three times per day for it to be effective. Taking less will likely not make much of a difference.

## 6. Different combinations produce different effects.

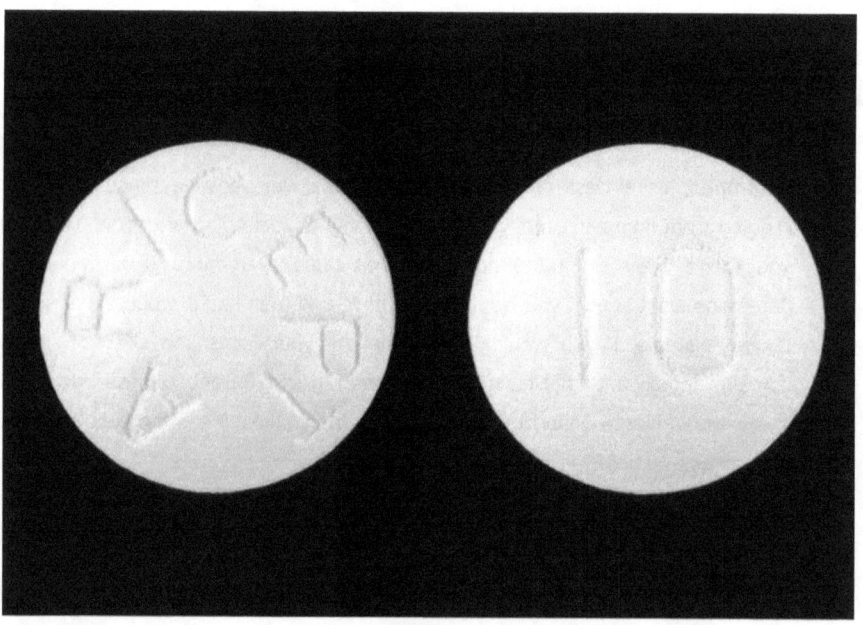

Nootropics are often combined into "stacks," a term that refers to when two or more nootropics are taken together to produce a specific effect. This helps customize the nootropics experience and users can choose the stack that will give them the desired results. Most users turn to nootropics to enhance their focus and concentration, and many stack combos aim to boost a user's motivation, mood, and memory. One important note: Certain nootropics are compounding, which means they are of stronger concentration, and, thus, the effects are more potent.

### 7. There are a variety of combinations.

As nootropics have become more popular, users have devised a practically endless variety of stack combinations. You can purchase pre-formulated stacks or create stacks on your own, although the pre-formulated stacks save the user considerable work since all of the dosings, measuring, weighing and mixing has already been done. Plus, for pre-formulated stacks, the final result has been proven to work, at least to some extent. Popular stack combos include L-theanine and caffeine, racetams or Noopept and choline, and St. John's-wort and ashwagandha. These are fairly basic combinations; many users employ more involved and advanced mixtures to achieve the desired effect.

### 8. They're intended for people with sleep disorders or cognitive issues.

Before they became trendy as "smart drugs," most nootropics were used for specific disorders. Many of these disorders were related to cognitive issues or sleep ailments. The nootropic drug Provigil (Modafinil), for instance, has long been prescribed by doctors for narcolepsy, shift-work sleep disorder, and chronic fatigue. Semax is often prescribed in Russia to treat ADHD and other hyperactivity conditions. Aricept (Donepezil) is a widely prescribed medication for treating and managing Alzheimer's disease.

## 9. Nootropic drugs are especially popular among college students.

It used to be that college students cramming for tests and aiming for optimum cognitive performance would depend on copious amounts of coffee to get through study sessions. Now, more and more are turning to nootropics to enhance and prolong the focus they feel they need. Though this spike in usage has not been without controversy, many students extol the virtues of nootropics for academic performance. A Swiss study found that as many as one in seven college students utilized nootropics for this purpose.

## 10.     Silicon Valley likes nootropics, too.

Nootropics are also extremely popular among the tech crowd of Silicon Valley. Given the hyper-focus needed for technical work like coding, computer folk seem to be the ideal market for nootropics. As a result, the nootropic industry in Silicon Valley is widely considered to be the most advanced and developed in the world. Tech entrepreneur George Burke told The Washington Post, "It's not like every tech worker in Silicon Valley is taking nootropics to get ahead. It's the few who are getting ahead who are using (nootropic) supplements to do that."

## 11.     The FDA does not approve some Nootropics.

The Food and Drug Administration approves not all nootropics, but that doesn't stop users from taking them. The FDA does not officially acknowledge the term nootropic, and the only approved versions are those used as prescription drugs such as Provigil and Aricept. Another popular nootropic called Piracetam is allegedly ideal for improving memory; however, it is not approved by the FDA. This means that any potential benefits or risks have not been sufficiently researched by the governing agency that oversees and regulates drugs and other substances--legal or otherwise. In other words: buyer beware.

**12.    Some users mix them with LSD microdoses or use LSD alone as a nootropic.**

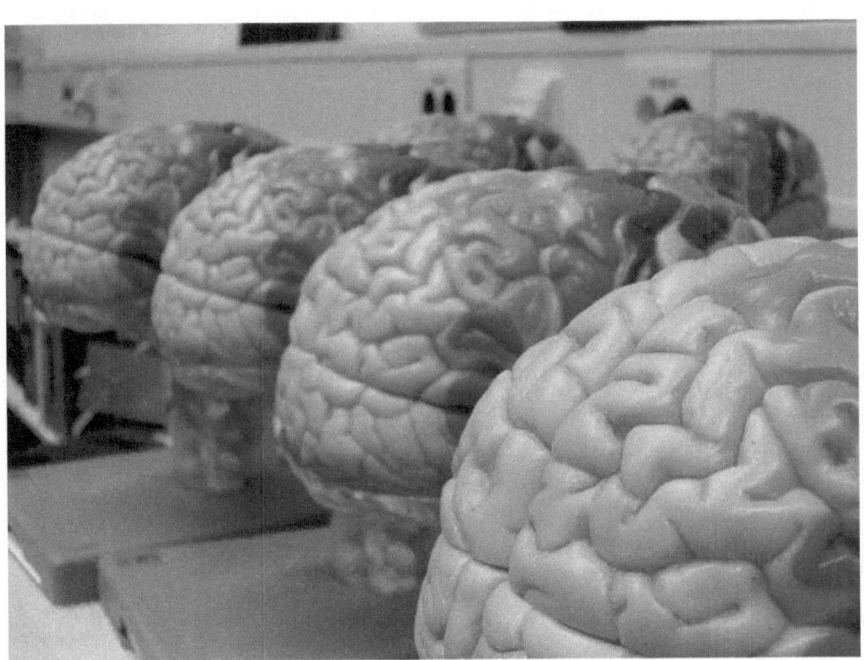

It's not uncommon for users to mix their nootropics with other substances like caffeine and nicotine (in supplement form, not smoky-smoky form). But one non-nootropic substance many are combining with their stacks is the '60s mainstay, LSD. This isn't the same dose you drop at the EDM festival. This dose is much smaller, and proponents say it mixes well with their nootropic stacks. Others use microdoses of LSD by itself.

## 13.     Regular use before age 25 could impair brain function.

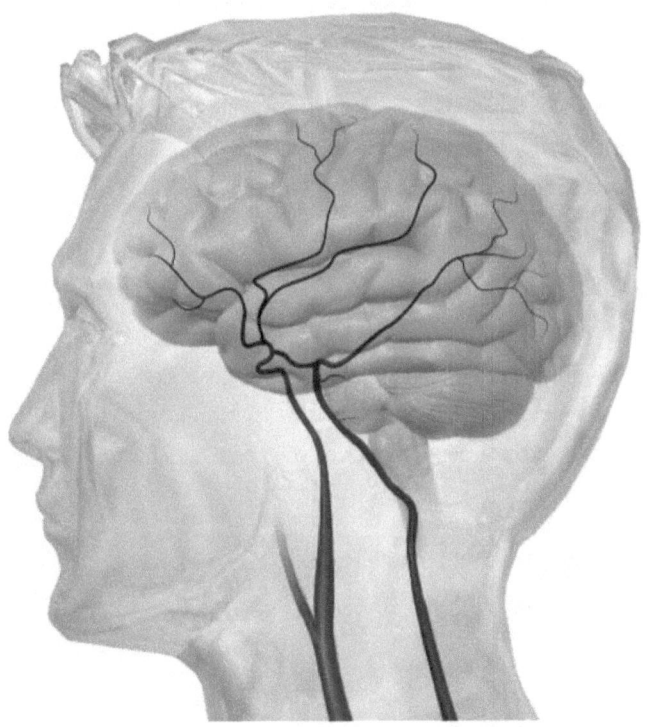

One of the mounting concerns surrounding nootropics is their use among young people, especially college students. Researchers believe that the human brain is not fully formed until 25 years old. This means that young people are changing their brain chemistry before their brains are even fully developed. Whether those changes are short- or long-term is not wholly understood yet. And that can be risky. Biological connections needed for healthy brain function are still maturing, and regular nootropic use could impair their development.

## 14. Building up tolerance is a possible issue.

One major area of discussion is whether one can build up a tolerance to nootropics. And, if so, what are the potential dangers of taking more to achieve the same effects? **According to Mental Health Daily:**

"Many people assume that tolerance cannot be established on nootropics, but I'd argue that they can. If you've had to increase your dose of a certain drug over some time to achieve the same effect, you've likely experienced some degree of tolerance. To minimize potential dangers, it is always recommended to take the 'minimal effective dose' or the amount that gives you benefit, without going overboard."

## 15. There isn't one single nootropic experience.

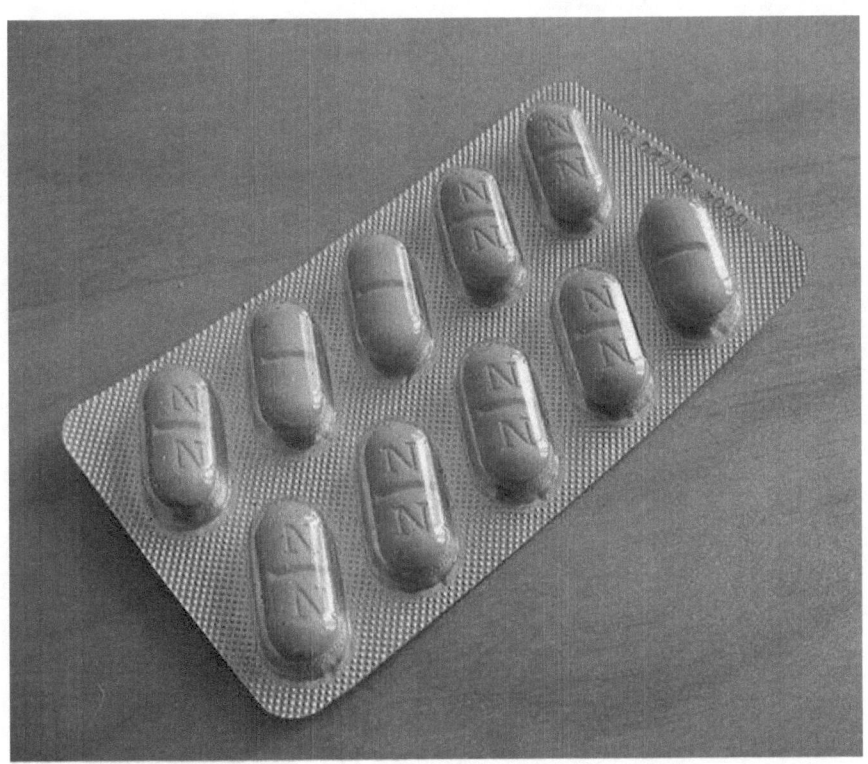

As with any drug, legal or otherwise, individual user experiences with nootropics can vary. The most commonly reported effects have to do with better focus and clarity but not every brain or body processes chemicals in the same way. Reactions can vary. Each nootropic has a different mechanism of action, meaning each one works differently on the brain. Experts suggest taking it slow when experimenting with nootropics, gauge your response and tweak your dosage as necessary.

## 16.     Nootropics can interact with other drugs.

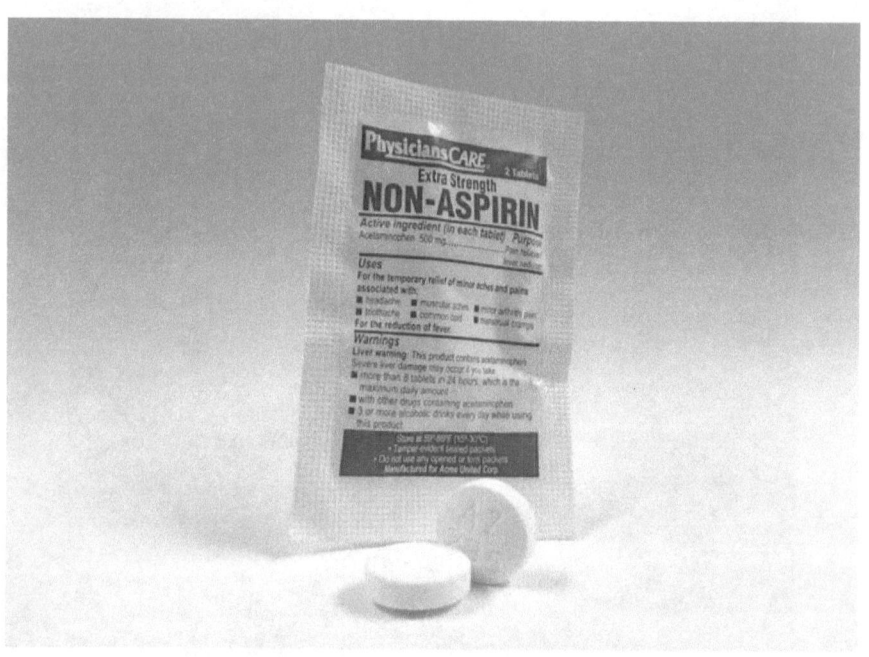

Researchers are also concerned by the ways nootropics can interact with other drugs. Some reactions can be ☐uite serious. Provigil (Modafinil), for example, can dangerously interfere with a variety of prescription drugs, mainly those prescribed for depression and ADHD, as well as benzodiazepines and blood thinners. Some over-the-counter meds can interact negatively with nootropics, too. The popular OTC pain reliever acetaminophen, for instance, is potentially hazardous when taking nootropics.

**17.      Many are illegal without a prescription, but legal to import.**

Several mainstream nootropics have been widely accepted and are perfectly legal; you need a doctor's prescription for a specific medical condition. But not everyone who uses nootropics, or wants to use nootropics, has a condition such as ADHD, narcolepsy, or Alzheimer's. So, they've turned to the internet to purchase nootropics without a prescription. Many are legal to import without a doctor's authorization. One example is the popular nootropic Piracetam, which cannot be obtained legally in the U.S. without a prescription, but is legal to import for personal use without one.

## 18. There's no shortage of nootropic horror stories and success stories.

Because different brains process different substances in different ways, nootropics have produced a wide range of experiences among users. Some have achieved positive results with nootropics, while others have had encounters that are nothing short of nightmares.

## 19. You can get smarter by consuming these drugs.

This is the most common misconception surrounding nootropics. While these drugs play no role in increasing your IQ level, they do offer various cognitive benefits, because of which, your mental performance is improved.

The benefits include increased focus, an increase in your overall attention span, enhanced learning functions, and better memory. With these drugs, you won't become smarter overnight, but you will feel more productive, focused, and motivated.

## 20.    The pills are unsafe.

Nootropics contain ingredients that have been approved by the FDA, and they are manufactured in facilities that are GMP certified. Thus, they adhere to □uality control measures, which mean that they are safe to use.

However, this doesn't mean that all nootropics available in the market, depending on the area, adhere to the □uality standards. While these aren't necessarily unsafe to consume, it is better if they are avoided.

Before you purchase a nootropic, it is better if you see if the □uality control and GMP certified logo is present on the pill or not. Also, you shouldn't alter the dose guidelines, or you might experience adverse effects.

## 21.    Nootropics are stimulants.

Some nootropics contain stimulants; however, this isn't the case always. Several stacks contain caffeine, but there is hardly any concern surrounding caffeine since it is a widely-consumed stimulant.

Numerous nootropics products don't contain caffeine or any other stimulant. Nootropics are known for providing cognitive enhancement and energy boosts, but the exact effects differ according to the product. There are hundreds of different kinds of nootropics, and each induces a different effect.

Some of the available nootropics reduce anxiety and stress while making the person feel relaxed and calm, without any increase in their energy. Meanwhile, other stacks are completely natural and are free from any kinds of stimulants.

## 22.     They are the same pills like the ones used in certain movies.

It has already been established that nootropics function as cognitive enhancers. By taking these pills, you can improve various cognitive functions such as mental energy, concentration, focus, memory, and learning.

But the effects that they produce aren't like the ones that the movie shows. Surely, you can't become a multimillionaire or a genius overnight just because you took such a pill. However, these pills indeed provide you with the edge that can help you to accomplish more.

## 23.     The pills are a cure for alzheimer's.

There are selected nootropic ingredients that have been commonly used for the treatment of Parkinson's, as well as Alzheimer's disease; however, nootropics themselves can't cure any of the two diseases.

Of course, a few of the nootropics can slow the cognitive decline that occurs because of old age. They can also improve memory function; thus, they are ☐uite beneficial for patients with Alzheimer's and Parkinson's. But a nootropic stack claiming to cure Alzheimer's is a promise that's quite unrealistic.

## 24. They must be cycled.

Manufacturers of a few nootropics suggest cycling the supplements so that the consumer doesn't develop a tolerance against the pills. However, this isn't always the case. Most of the nootropics can be used continuously without cycling or a break. Still, it is better to follow the instructions given with each supplement.

## 25. There are no side effects.

A lot of brain pills have no side effects, but the same can't be said about nootropics. Different ingredients, when taken in different dosages, induce varying effects. Each person might experience a different side effect.

By definition, nootropics aren't toxic. However, because of the body chemistry, it is advised to start with the lowest dosage that has been recommended and then increase the dose slowly.

If you are new to nootropics, then it is better to start with some of the safer nootropics that have been used for a long time now. Examples of such nootropics include L-Theanine and Bacopa Monnieri. Since these are natural nootropics, they have been used for years in traditional medicine and are the best option.

While some nootropics include a warning of mild effects like an upset stomach or headaches, others might cause serious side effects.

### 26.    They are a replacement for quality sleep, proper nutrition, and hard work.

You might want to rely on these pills to bring you success. But the reality is completely different. Just like other supplements, nootropics also produce the best results when they are combined with a productive and healthy lifestyle.

Like you can't expect to shed a few pounds by taking a weight loss supplement and eating as much junk food you want, you also can't expect nootropics to give you the push you need to pull off a successful all-nighter.

So, to reap the maximum benefits from these nootropics pill, you must eat healthily, stay active, and get sufficient sleep.

### 27.    If you don't experience a change, then the pill isn't working.

You shouldn't expect to experience any effect right after you have consumed the first supplement. There might be some rare reviews of nootropics that provide an immediate effect; however, you must know that nootropics react differently in each individual.

Every human being's body chemistry is uni□ue from the next person. The body chemistry has a big impact on how the body absorbs substances and metabolizes.

While a few people might undergo the pill's effects just within fifteen minutes, it isn't necessary that you would do too. However, this also doesn't mean that you should give up. Some nootropics need time to get used to your system before producing any effects.

Try out the supplement for a month at least, before changing it and trying out a new nootropic.

## 28.     Nootropics only work short term.

Many nootropics have been backed up by research, which proves that they work for the long term. One example is Bacopa Monnieri, which has been proved to improve the cognitive function for 12 weeks.

However, since funding multi-year studies on nootropics aren't easy, there is hardly any research which studies the effect of nootropics beyond a year. It can be surely said that many nootropics can easily work for more than one year until tolerance occurs inside the body.

### 29.    Nootropics can give you a super-human brain boost, like in the movies.

For better or for worse, none of the legal or well-researched nootropic herbs, compounds, or supplement available on the market today can give you superpowers – despite what any Hollywood blockbusters may suggest.

Keeping that in mind, research has found that certain nootropic ingredients, compounds, stacks, and supplements may be capable of supporting factors like focus, energy, mood, and overall productivity.

### 30.    The right nootropic can help you find a shortcut to success/achieving your goals.

Not exactly. Just like every other type of nutritional supplement on the market today, nootropic supplements are never designed or intended to replace key aspects of an individual's routine or lifestyle – this includes everything from good sleeping habits and a healthy diet to hard-work and dedication.

That said, there's a healthy body of scientific research suggesting that the benefits that may come with nootropic supplementation can have the potential to aid an individual trying to achieve certain tasks and goals.

### 31.    All nootropics provide the same benefits.

While there's no denying that almost all of the researched and recognized benefits of nootropics are linked to cognitive health in one way or another, nootropics may offer supplement takers an impressive variety of benefits.

Acknowledging that it's not uncommon for the effects and experience with a given nootropic to vary slightly from individual to individual, studies and research have linked a "family" of potential benefits and effects to ingredients and supplement that have been categorized as a nootropic in nature.

Some of the most researched and common benefits (and potential benefits) of nootropic supplements have come to **include the support of:**

- Memory
- Energy levels and mood
- Focus
- Reasoning
- Creativity

Different ingredients, ingredient variations, and ingredient combinations are poised to provide different results. Finding the right nootropic for a given need can be as simple as doing some research. That said, when considering the addition of a new supplement to a routine – nootropic or otherwise – individuals are always advised to seek professional medical or nutritional guidance.

## 32.    All nootropics are relatively new, under-researched, and synthetic.

This last myth couldn't be further from the truth. While it is true that a number of popular nootropic ingredients reuire a degree of processing and distillation in order to be viable and that there are others that only came into being during the 20th century, there are just as many (if not more) ingredients with "natural" origins and long-standing histories of human use.

Certain plant-based nootropics, like ginseng and Bacopa monnieri, have centuries' worth of anecdotal evidence supporting their viability as well as impressive collections of modern scientific research supporting their potential benefits and efficacy.

## 33.    Are nootropics a Limitless pill?

Not exactly. The film Limitless popularized smart drugs and cognitive enhancement, but this is an exaggerated depiction. Any attempt to sell a Limitless pill is a marketing attempt to separate you from your hard-earned money.

## 34.    Are stimulants (like Adderall) nootropics?

Not really. While Adderall and similarly strong stimulants can improve focus and concentration, many studies suggest they harm cognitive function.

## 35.    Are nootropics snake oil?

It depends. Most individual compounds (such as creatine, piracetam, or bacopa) have more research than blended nootropics (such as Alpha Brain or CILTEP). Many of the nootropic compounds work in theory and practice, but many products are way too expensive and do not provide any profound effects.

## 36.     Are nootropics legal?

Most nootropics are legal to use or considered in a legal gray area. It is considered illegal to use drugs like modafinil without a prescription in some countries, but there is little evidence of government organizations carrying out any criminal activity.

## 37.     Are nootropics safe?

Every nootropic has a relatively safe dosage range to start, but each unique person will react with chemical compounds differently. One safe way to start would be to use the Alexander Shulgin method. You take a fraction of a total dose to rule out allergy, then half dose to rule out negative reactions, and finally take a full recommended dosage.

## 38.     Do nootropics work long term?

Yes. Many nootropics have research to indicate that they work long-term. Bacopa monnieri is one example, which is known to improve cognitive function for at least 12 weeks. Unfortunately, funding multi-year nootropic studies is not easy, so there are few studies beyond one year. It is plausible to say many nootropics work long-term beyond one year, however.

### 39.    How do I know if nootropics are working?

Many nootropics will come with a distinct "feeling", which is often subjective and hard to ☐uantify. Although many beginners to nootropics desire to have felt from smart drugs, not all of them will. Some of the most well-researched nootropics (such as creatine or bacopa) will likely provide no subjective "feeling" at all.

Tracking the subjective feeling via a journal will help you to understand better how nootropics impact you. Another method is to use cognitive tests and metrics such as Quantified Mind and Cambridge Brain Sciences.

### 40.    Any one of any age can use them.

It is a false belief that any smart drug or nootropic work with anyone of any age but the truth is some nootropics work maximally with and for younger people while others work well with aging brains.

### 41.    You will get an instant gratification.

This is another fact that needs to be debunked. As a beginner in the consumption of nootropics, it could erroneously be thought that after the fast dosage one gets to feel 'something' immediately, but this might not be the case for everyone though.

To get a great and full result of a smart drug, be disciplined to stay with one for at least one month.

## 42. They do not give a sense of euphoria.

At the beginning of the user's dosage, one is left feeling high morally, but a slight miscalculation regarding the use of a particular nootropic could lead you to an end that was not expected or anticipated. These seemingly 'harmless' smart drugs can lead and leave someone hallucinating and ⬜uite euphoric.

## 43. They are fad.

Another fact about nootropics is that they are the 'in thing' now. This is not a fact or the truth. For many thousand years past, Adaptogens (natural/herbal drugs that enhance and help the body adapt from stress to focus), have been used as major memory boosters or enhancers. For instance, Ashwagandha is one of such Adaptogens which has been used in India as a traditional drug as a cognitive booster, and it is still being used widely. Piracetam is another smart drug or nootropic found in the early 60s and still being used up to date.

## 44. They are only for disability free individuals.

Another widespread belief about nootropics is that it can only work when your thinking faculties are soberly working but just fatigued due to pressure or stress. This may sound and even look true, but it is so far from the truth. Studies show that moderate usage or dosage of the smart drug Piracetam by dyslexic students on a very regular pattern would trigger off understanding and analytical skills.

## 45. You can start using the drugs whenever you wish and at any time.

As a beginner in the utilization of these smart drugs, it is assumed that is it okay to start using any drug for enhancement, but that is not the right thing to do. You should not go that direction.  Instead, start using lighter and relatively safer nootropic like herbals in small dosages daily.  How about starting with bulletproof coffee? You can also start with only one nootropic before you jump to designing a stack for yourself.  If you are highly convinced about using a stack of nootropics, then go for a pre-formulated stack.

## 46. As long as you use nootropics, you do not have to keep up with healthy living.

No matter how packed your work schedule could be, living on coffee, most of the days is not the best way to go in the □uest of saving time to work. You must be careful of relying on smart drugs for enhancement of performance because, at a point, this might go wrong or backfire. Nootropics or smart drugs must never be a replacement for a healthy living, which includes enough sleep, exercise, and a healthy standard eating pattern.

## 47. Nootropics are backed up with scientific evidence.

There is a lot of talks around nootropics, also known as smart drugs that could convince you that there is strong scientific evidence to back up the practicality of these drugs. This has led to the reason why a huge number of people are jumping over them even though a lot is yet to be known or discovered on how much a nootropic impacts the brain. There is a lot that is left to be desired scientifically.

## 48.      You will be a success in a blink of an eye.

If you are looking for a shortcut towards success by using this drug, then you are in for a big disappointment. Nootropics are not charms or magic drugs that perform miracles. They work in a process and over a period. Using nootropics regularly would surely enhance your memory, improve your vitality and even help your focus on any endeavor more intently but these will not automatically make you a millionaire of a sort of a genius from nowhere just like that. Let no one lie to you to convince you of purchasing the drug.

## 49.      You use 10% of your brain.

Nootropics don't help you to use more than 10% of the brain because all humans use every part of the brain. Cognition occurs via pathways and the connections between them. The more connections you have, the better your cognition and memory, and you can certainly add neural pathways or improve existing ones.

Learning a new skill will add new connections. So will learning new ways of focusing or using memory. Nootropics can also enhance neuroplasticity in a huge number of ways by improving blood flow to the brain. That said, the brain is a complex organ, and much of its functionality isn't entirely understood. Sometimes neuroscientists can't produce reasons for the effects they observe.

## 50. Nootropics are adequate replacements for nutrition and hard work.

Nutrients keep your cells healthy. Without them, even the most effective nootropics will have little effect on your cognition. Before you build a house, you create the foundation. Otherwise, the entire structure will collapse. The same applies to your health. First, you must lay the foundation with good nutrition that contributes to your cellular health. It's only then that other medications can be at their most effective. A wholesome and healthy diet is one of the most important elements of your brain's health. Deficiencies can obliterate your ability to function.

- Iron deficiency can cause fatigue and weakness. 30% of the world has this problem.
- Thiamine deficiency chips away at your energy levels and memory.
- Niacin deficiency causes dementia.
- Folate deficiency reduces brain development and impedes a healthy nervous system.

# Chapter 7

## What Are Nootropics?

Smart drugs are the common name for nootropics. What are they used for? Quite simply, they are used to increase our bodies' supply of brain functionality. This brain functionality is done through the brain's neurotransmitters. Nootropics also boost up the brain's enzymes and hormones, as well as kick up the oxygen supply and growing more nerves, and being as there are deficient levels of toxicity if any at all, it is next to impossible for anyone to overdose on nootropic substances. On top of this, side effects are slim to none, and in fact, many nootropic substances work better together.

A majority of nootropics are simple nutrients or plant parts like roots, herbs or bark. You can get these nootropic substances over the counter at your grocery or health food store, and you can find them in most nutritional supplements. Some nootropics are classified as drugs, that are part of the treatment for retardation, Alzheimer's and Parkinson's.

Working to support your brain's neurotransmitters, and keeping them at high levels, will reward you with increased abilities in the area of concentration, creativity, mood, recall, memory encoding, calculation ability, and mental focus. Nootropics are even used to prevent and cure most forms of depression.

The thing about thinking that most people will not find hard to believe is that it is not easy. When the neurotransmitters fire off all the neurons needed for the brain to work, the supply is run down. If the supply isn't replenished, then you will start to experience slower mental processing, a hard time concentrating, difficulty reasoning, and you will find learning to be more difficult. Additionally, your recall will suffer, as will your coordination, and you will find your moods hanging out somewhere near the bottom. You will find it hard to cope with.

You can see that nootropics are crucial to your brainpower, especially as you get older. Having the ability to enhance your brain's own ability to function at its highest level should give you comfort. The biggest fear of getting older is losing the ability to think, reason and recall. No one wants to lose the ability to function in society. By spending your life developing a regimen that includes exercise and nootropics, you can face your golden years with a golden mind. As with any nutritional supplement, you will want to discuss your intentions with your doctor and nutritionist.

**Nootropic Ingredients**

If you're looking to dip your toes into the world of nootropics and boost brain performance, including natural nootropics in your wellness routine is the way to go. These can be easily accessed, and you'd be surprised by how many you are probably already familiar with.

- **Caffeine**

Everyone's favorite, caffeine is the superstar nootropic. Found in coffee, green tea, and chocolate, chances are you've been using this for your morning boost for years. You can also find caffeine supplements if you aren't a fan of any of the usual vehicles. Caffeine helps you feel more alert and wakes you up by blocking your brain's adenosine receptors.

- **L-Theanine**

If caffeine alone isn't cutting it, add in this amino acid to boost the benefits of both of these nootropics. L-theanine and caffeine are both naturally occurring in tea, especially green tea, making this beverage the better choice over coffee if you want the boost of both, with studies showing the combination of these two resulted in faster reaction time and improved mental fatigue.

- **Creatine**

This amino acid is used by your body to make protein and promote muscle growth, making it a popular supplement among athletes. It is also considered great fuel for your brain because it binds with phosphate in your brain to give energy to your brain's cells for increased short-term memory.

- **Gingko Biloba**

You can't expect me to get through a list of herbs without mentioning at least one adaptogen. The leaves of the ginkgo Biloba tree are a powerful brain booster. Not only has this been shown to improve memory, but it can also alleviate stress by decreasing your stress hormone, cortisol.

- **Panax ginseng**

This other superstar adaptogen works to improve memory by reducing oxidative stress to promote brain-protecting nitric oxide. Research has further shown this adaptogen's brain-boosting power with its ability to prevent age-related memory loss and improve long-term memory.

- **Curcumin**

You may have 99 problems, but curcumin has probably already solved 98 of them—and you can add improved cognitive performance to that list. This compound in turmeric has been shown to improve working memory with consistent long-term supplementation. Curcumin can also increase BDNF, reduce oxidative stress, and inhibit inflammatory cytokines.

- **Bacopa**

Bacopa monnieri is a nootropic herb that has been used in traditional medicine for longevity and cognitive enhancement. Supplementation has been shown to reduce anxiety and improve memory formation.

- **Rhodiola**

Rhodiola Rosea is a plant whose roots are known to have "adaptogenic" properties helping the body handle stress. Rhodiola is most commonly used for increasing energy, endurance, strength, and mental capacity. Preliminary research shows it to have neuroprotective and anti-inflammatory benefits.

- **Pycnogenol**

Pine bark extract is one of nature's super antioxidants. It's loaded with oligomeric proanthocyanidin compounds (OPCs) which possess antibacterial, antiviral, anticarcinogenic, anti-aging, anti-inflammatory and anti-allergic properties.

- **Omega 3's**

Fish oil and krill oil are the most common types of omega-3 fat supplements. Omega-3fatty acids play important roles in brain function and development. In addition to many health benefits throughout your body, omega-3 supplementation has been shown to reduce anxiety and depression, reduce symptoms of ADHD in children, improve psychiatric disorders, and fight age-related mental decline and Alzheimer's disease. One study even found that people who eat fatty fish had more gray matter in the brain and improved memory.

**Why take nootropics?**

Nootropics are brain enhancers or cognitive enhancers. They work by enhancing the brain's ability to function better. Nootropics are made from synthetic and natural substances, which increases blood flow to the brain, makes the neurotransmitter signals work better, and helps the brain work much more efficiently and smartly. Since there comes the need to compete, perform, and outrun other competitive minds in many cases, nootropics are a great help. If you know well how to take smart drugs, and healthily assimilate them into your busy life, so that you get their help when you need the most, then you can make way through various situations with a smartly performing brain.

**The main benefits of nootropics are:**

- They help improve memory.
- Aids in learning.
- Damaging degenerative diseases of the brain like Alzheimer's, Parkinson's, and Huntington's can be avoided and blocked with the use of smart drugs.
- They increase your hours of wakefulness, and you don't feel sleepy by taking them.
- If you restrict the consumption of smart drugs to a healthy threshold limit, then they are not toxic and does not interfere with health.
- The fogginess in mind gets clear and removed with them, and you can think better, act better, and altogether, performance gets enhanced.
- You don't feel fatigued mentally soon while working on a brain-racking project.

Other benefits which are observed **along with it are:**

- Anxiety levels are lessened
- Energy gets boosted
- The aging of the brain is delayed which contributes to overall longevity

**When should you take smart drugs?**

The effect of nootropics on the brain is a sudden boost of extra energy, more awareness about your surroundings, objects, problems and solutions, better understanding, a highly alert mental state with full wakefulness and a much better power to concentrate. These are the immediate effects of having a smart drug. There are some good long-term effects too, which are not felt by you directly but found through scientific researches. Degenerative diseases of the brain are slowed or prevented to a huge extent when you take smart drugs. However, nootropics must not be taken regularly, although if you take them daily, it will not cause any adverse effects. To be sure, you should not take even natural substances every day to avoid the chances of addiction or habit-forming. They are to be taken only when you need it. The good news is researched on nootropics have revealed that they are safe for use, and are non-toxic in optimum doses, and also do not form a habit.

This means, when you know you have to give in more than you do normally in a day, then you need the smart drugs. If you are wakeful for a certain period, and on a certain day, for some serious work, you want to increase your wakefulness and alertness, then you need to take a nootropic. With the effect of a nootropic, you would be able to give in undivided attention into something you want to and work with extreme focus and alertness without getting the brain fatigue to feel. And this feeling lasts for a full 24 hours. This means, what you get for a few hours with a couple of cups of coffee, you get that in full with a single dose of a nootropic.

## How nootropics help in reducing brain fog?

A foggy brain is what makes you sometimes slow in thinking, confused in taking decisions, unable to work and concentrate, unable to think deep, and also a little dumb or low in situations. If you are experiencing any such thing, then you may get more alert and active, and feel that you are giving in more than you would normally with the help of a nootropic. There are many reasons behind a foggy brain. It may be inade☐uate sleep, lack of exercise, a bad diet and deficiency in nutrients, and many other factors. But the brain gets the power to work with full force when it gets a good supply of blood. Blood carries oxygen to the brain cells, and also gives enough energy. That is why the brain can function better, when a smart drug triggers the flow of blood in good amount to the brain, to help it function great.

## Get good memory with nootropics.

Experience a great boost in memory with nootropics too. Bad or poor memory is the result of lack of sleep, bad diet, stress, etc. With smart drugs, this problem can be solved to quite an extent. The drug will be able to give you brain the much-needed balanced nutrients delivered so that the brain can function better, and memory also gets enhanced. In any case, it has been seen that smart drugs also reduce inflammation in the brain, and helps avoid chances of Alzheimer's disease.

# Conclusion

Piracetam is a synthetic nootropic that may boost mental performance. Its positive effects on the brain seem more apparent in older adults, as well as people with mental impairment, dementia, or learning disorders, such as dyslexia. That said, very few studies on piracetam exist, and most of the research is dated, so new research is needed before it can be recommended.

Piracetam is relatively safe for most people. Still, if you're taking medication or have any medical disorders, speak to your healthcare provider before trying this drug.

If you get to know the real facts about Nootropics, you would know that they are friendly drugs, which are to give you great power and productivity for great output, and then you may use them accordingly for a better career and studies.

are turning Science into a dogma, as you thoroughly believe, especially when the public act takes place, all you spent so much time writing is 100% correct. That same day, in a country far away, where the time zone is ahead of your own, someone else might be proving you wrong. It does not have to be the next day, it could be simultaneously.

All of this to say we do not speak the absolute truth. There are some things in life we have come to learn are not questionable, but only until they are, preferably with sustainable arguments, without raising doubts for no good reason. This book could be brilliant to some, valid to others, invalid to some others from a series of different points of view or, ultimately, ridiculous as can be. Either way, they (whoever they are) do not prevent me from speaking my mind, and neither should you allow others to do the same to you. The real Utopia is made of democratic plurality to all, and not to an isolated elite, deciding what becomes public or forever forgotten.

My best to you and thank you for allowing me to keep you company, through my words and thoughts, across this reading journey.

# Bonus Round

# «Brexit»: a Path to Dystopia

On Thursday, June 23rd, 2016, the United Kingdom of Great Britain and Northern Ireland and Gibraltar[352] voted a referendum which became known as «Brexit» within the media and «EU Referendum» among the country's nationals, though it is formally addressed to as the «United Kingdom European Union Membership Referendum». The question asked in the voting ballot was:

«Should the United Kingdom remain a member of the European Union or leave the European Union?».

The right to abandon the EU has been possible ever since the Treaty of Lisbon[353] was signed by all Member-States. Article 50

---

[352] A British Overseas Territory under the former's administration since the beginning of the 18th century.

[353] Signed on December 13th, 2007 and applicable since December 1st, 2009. It is an amendment to the Maastricht Treaty of 1992, which created the EU as the successor to the European Economic Community, and the Treaty of Rome of 1958, which founded the EEC. Its complete designation is «Treaty

is the one setting the necessary procedures for withdrawal of a Member-State from the EU. It reads:

«1. Any Member-State may decide to withdraw from the Union in accordance with its own constitutional requirements.

2. A Member-State which decides to withdraw shall notify the European Council of its intention. In the light of the guidelines provided by the European Council, the Union shall negotiate and conclude an agreement with that State, setting out the arrangements for its withdrawal, taking account of the framework for its future relationship with the Union. That agreement shall be negotiated in accordance with Article 218(3)[354] of the Treaty on the Functioning of the European Union. It shall be concluded on behalf of the Union by the Council, acting by a qualified majority, after obtaining the consent of the European Parliament.

3. The Treaties shall cease to apply to the State in question from the date of entry into force of the withdrawal agreement or, failing that, two years after the notification referred to in paragraph 2, unless the European Council, in agreement with the Member-State concerned, unanimously decides to extend this period».

At the time this «Bonus Round» is being produced for later playing, beginning September 2016, the UK has *not* begun the negotiation process comprising its withdrawal from the EU.

---

of Lisbon amending the Treaty on European Union and the Treaty establishing the European Community».

[354] «3. The Commission, or the High Representative of the Union for Foreign Affairs and Security Policy where the agreement envisaged relates exclusively or principally to the common foreign and security policy, shall submit recommendations to the Council, which shall adopt a decision authorizing the opening of negotiations and, depending on the subject of the agreement envisaged, nominating the Union negotiator or the head of the Union's negotiating team».

Political analysts from all over the world have stated the Prime-Minister under whose Government the referendum took place, David Cameron[355], is the one to be held responsible for this event, as it was one of the electoral promises he said he would keep in order to be reelected in the 2015 General Election, though he always campaigned against the withdrawal.

During the campaign, Member of Parliament Jo Cox[356], who was pro-European, was brutally murdered on the street (shot and stabbed multiple times) in Birstall, West Yorkshire, in broad daylight, by 52-year-old local Thomas Mair, who was charged with murder and other offenses, namely the stabbing and injuring of 77-year-old Bernard Carter-Kenny, who tried to fight Mair away from Cox, though his rescue attempt could not save her.

You would think such a senseless killing (as any killing is) would make voters choose the first part of the question in the voting ballot, but the majority chose indeed to leave the EU. Those campaigning for the withdrawal were mainly Nigel Farage[357], leader of the UK Independence Party, a position he quit from on July 4th, 2016, and Boris Johnson[358], former Mayor of London and Secretary of State for Foreign and Commonwealth Affairs under Theresa May[359], who has since July 13th, 2016 become the second female Prime Minister of the UK[360], following David Cameron's resignation, even though he only planned to leave in October.

Statistics reveal the British youth who voted wanted to stay in the European Union, whereas elderly citizens wanted to definitely

---

[355] B. 1966.
[356] 1974-2016.
[357] B. 1964.
[358] Idem.
[359] B. 1956.
[360] The first was Baroness Margaret Thatcher (1925-2013), also known as «Iron Lady». She assumed office between 1979 and 1990.

leave and gain back their independence, even though Prime-Minister Cameron had negotiated with the EU ever since his reelection a privileged membership, stating a few conditions such as never accepting to be a part of the Eurozone or salvaging countries in the vicinity of bankruptcy within said organization. No matter how hard he tried to campaign for the Pro-European policy, Mr. Cameron eventually triggered nationalist movements in Britain that politicians like Mr. Farage and Mr. Johnson took advantage of, though neither of them wanted to stay on the ship as it foundered.

Curiously enough, Donald Trump[361], US presidential hopeful under the Republican Party, was in Scotland the following weekend, taking the Scottish example as an inspiration to his own objectives back to his homeland. The misinformed candidate was bludgeoned harshly on social media, namely Twitter, by British nationals who made him realize Scotland had voted to stay in the EU, as much as Northern Ireland and Gibraltar, opposed by England and Wales.

Obviously, what is now the United Kingdom may soon crumble apart, as Scottish Prime-Minister Nicola Sturgeon[362] has considered the possibility of a new referendum regarding Scotland's presence in the Kingdom. Back in September 2014, the country voted to stay with London when asked whether it should become an independent nation, especially for fear of investment withdrawals in its territory. Now, the political and economic paradigms are entirely different. It is not just Scotland that is at a loss, but rather the entire UK.

Because «Brexit» is a non-binding referendum under British law, it does not mean its resolution should have to be approved by Parliament. However, and traditionally, when the British people are asked something regarding their future as a nation, their

---

[361] B. 1946.
[362] B. 1970.

will is respected, even if that same will is only approved by a very small majority, which was the case (51.89% against 48.11%).

After Britain and the rest of the world came to know the referendum results, nationalists across Europe were eager to loosen their tongue in favor of a similar referendum voted by their respective countries, which are also a part of the EU, namely Belgium, France, Germany, Hungary, Italy, Poland, Spain and Sweden. The first two countries listed above are the very heart of the EU, and yet they would not say no to holding a referendum on withdrawal from the Union, registering dangerous percentages toward leaving[363].

We are either before a repetitive simulation, or we are undoubtedly living in stupidity, driving the people toward the support of one person's (the leader of each nationalist party in Europe) political ambitions. Nationalism across Europe seems to be cyclical and, subsequently, disruptive. Those who are forced to fight against anyone threatening the freedom of their nation eventually grow old and die happy for having saved their fellow countrymen from tyranny, especially those who will be born beyond it. It is these people, who have always been in contact with freedom and Democracy, that end up craving for a national identity, unknowing the consequences of such a thought out of their own experience. The time they live in is one thing, the time before them is another.

It only proves to me that nationalism, who some people are led to think is a good thing for them and their country, in order to keep its sovereignty among others, is precisely the kind of disease that keeps festering and cannot be completely annihilated

---

[363] AKKOC, Raziye, 05-10-2016, *The Telegraph*, «How Brexit could lead to other EU countries following the UK out», (http://www.telegraph.co.uk/news/2016/05/09/how-brexit-could-lead-to-other-eu-countries-following-the-uk-out/), accessed 07-19-2016. Though this article was written previously to the referendum, it was already making sense.

from the face of the Earth, just like garden weeds. That is why, so as to keep the timeline closer to the present, there was a World War I, followed by a World War II, nearly twenty years later.

There was a sleeper war for over forty years, the Cold War, though there were several others in the middle, constantly involving the United States, who somehow agreed upon the idea they had a mission to become the world's police, spreading Democracy at whatever the cost, enabling the formation of terrorist cells in the Middle East, who began their revenge against America a long time ago, making Europe pay the price as well, because of NATO.

No one goes to war for the sake of a faith or any other cause. Far beyond that, there is always a national, political and economic interest behind it. The problem is the kind of interest topping all others: the individual.

# Biography

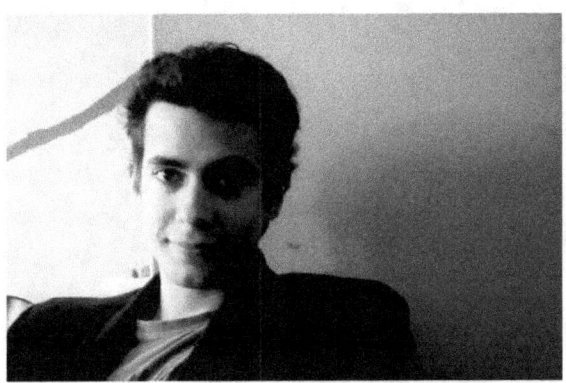

Tiago Lameiras was born in Lisbon, Portugal, in 1990.

He has a Bachelor's Degree on Theater – Acting, taken at the Higher School of Theater and Film of Lisbon.

He is currently completing the PhD on Communications, Culture and Arts – Cultural Studies Specialization, at the Faculty of Human and Social Science of the University of the Algarve, Portugal.

He also has among several publications titles of his own, such as *Portvcale – A Epopeia Portuguesa da Contemporaneidade* (October 2010), *Viagem ao Centro de Ti – Romance Trovado* (January 2012), *A Mão de Diónisos* (November 2013) and *Actor Being: A Role in Mankind* (March 2016), as well as poetical collaborations in Chiado Editora's Poetry Anthologies *Entre o Sono e o Sonho* (2012, 2014 and 2015) and Sinapsis' *Enigma(s)* (February 2015).